The Forgotten Trimester: Navigating Self-Care After Birth

By Megan Gray, MD

Table of Contents

Introduction

Pregnancy is an exciting time! We spend 10 months watching our bellies grow in great anticipation for the new life to come. The major focus of attention by our physicians, family and friends is our health as we move through the three trimesters of pregnancy. We count down the trimesters, the months, the weeks, and the days until finally he or she is here: your wonderfully beautiful miracle. Then you take baby home and naturally, the focus becomes baby. *Throughout the whirlwind of the first 12 weeks of baby's arrival home, we tend to neglect the importance of the next three to four months of our own life...the fourth trimester.*

I believe that the first three months after delivery set the tone for your relationship with your child and your expanding family. As I navigated my own postpartum course, *I realized how neglected the first 12 weeks after delivery truly becomes.* I noticed there is a lack of supportive, valid information for women navigating postpartum. Not until I went through it personally did I realize that as an obstetrician, I had not been giving the fourth trimester the attention it deserves for my patients.

My hope for this book is to provide a source of guidance for one of the most important, yet often overlooked moments in time, the fourth trimester. This time involves a rollercoaster of emotions from ultimate bliss, to utter frustration, exhaustion, and anxiety. The combination of rapidly changing hormones, lack of sleep, body changes and the responsibility of a new life are all a part of the rollercoaster. This book is meant to be a quick reference to help you take care of yourself during this very busy time, so you can confidently spend most of your time enjoying your new baby and your new life!

This book is not meant to be exhaustive and does not include everything you may experience in the fourth trimester, but I have included the most common concerns and complaints I had as a patient and those I hear as a physician. It is designed so that you can rapidly flip to an issue and be reassured. This book is not a replacement for guidance by your physician or lactation consultant. Listen to your body – you are your best healthcare advocate and if something does not seem right to you, then contact your physician. Wishing the best of luck to you and your new family!

Chapter 1: Going Home – The Basics

You probably have a laundry list of items that you need at home for baby, but do you know what you need to take care of yourself for the first few days to weeks after you bring baby home? Listed are a few items you should have at your disposal.

What you will need:

    1. **Pads**: I recommend full-sized, thick pads that are fragrance free for the first two weeks after delivery. You will probably be able to switch to a thinner panty liner after two weeks as your vaginal bleeding becomes lighter.

2. **Perineal cleansing bottle (peri-bottle):** This looks like an empty shampoo bottle. It is used to cleanse the perineum and vagina throughout the day.

Most hospitals will give you a peri-bottle you can take home with you after delivery. If you did not get one of these at the hospital, you can purchase them online for less than $5. In addition to cleansing your bottom, *you can also use the bottle filled with tap water to dilute urine as you are voiding to reduce the pain with urination.*

3. **Ice packs:** You can either purchase ice packs from a sports store or drugstore, or you can make them at home with Ziploc bags and ice. You can also take a diaper, cut open the top and fill the middle with ice. It will absorb the water as the ice melts and has a soft inner liner, so you don't have to wrap it prior to placing against your skin.

-Use ice packs to reduce the soreness and swelling of the perineum after delivery.

-Never place ice packs directly against the skin; instead, wrap in a thin towel or old T-shirt before applying against the skin.

-Apply lightly wrapped ice packs to the skin for 15-20 minutes, three to four times daily.

4. **Sitz bath basin**: This is a shallow basin that can fit over your toilet. I prefer this over a bath tub because it takes less water to fill it up so you can use it on the fly – a must when you have a newborn – and it is easier to clean between uses (imagine cleaning your bath tub every time you use it for a sitz bath...umm no, you won't have time for that!). You can fill these shallow basins with two to three inches of warm (not hot) tap water to soak your bottom. Avoid adding soap, bubble bath or salts to the water. Be sure to clean the basin well and dry well between uses.

5. **Dermoplast:** This is an over-the-counter pain-relieving spray containing a numbing agent, benzocaine. You can spray this directly on your bottom as needed after a vaginal delivery to help relieve perineal discomfort.

6. **Stool softener**: Keeping your bowel movements soft will prevent the need for straining. This will reduce stress on your vaginal sutures if you had a vaginal tear or an episiotomy. If you had a C-section, use stool softeners to avoid straining with bowel movements to make bathroom time less painful. Colace, Miralax, Dulcolax – all of which are okay to use while breast-feeding – are stool softeners you can purchase at your local drugstore without a prescription.

7. **Comfortable loose-fitting clothes**: Sorry ladies, you won't be wearing your skinny jeans home from the hospital. Avoid tight-fitting undergarments and pants to allow for the perineum to breathe. Cotton undergarments are best to allow for airflow and wicking away of moisture.

8. **Breast pads**: If you are breast-feeding, these pads will protect nipples and prevent leaking of milk onto clothing. There are disposable, single use breast pads or reusable, washable breast pads. This is personal preference. If you choose the reusable breast pads, be sure

to wash them frequently with a mild laundry detergent and allow them to dry completely prior to use.

9. **Lanolin ointment**: If you are breast-feeding, this product helps to prevent dry, cracked and painful nipples. You can start using the lanolin ointment immediately; you don't have to wait until you have symptoms. Apply ointment to nipples after each feed. This product is nontoxic and does not have to be removed prior to feeding baby.

10. **Nursing bra**: If you are breast-feeding, invest in a few good nursing bras. These bras allow for quick and easy access while nursing your newborn.

11. **Prenatal vitamins**: Don't forget to continue your prenatal vitamins daily if you are breast-feeding.

12. **Breast pump/breast pump parts** – Currently, most insurance companies provide women with a breast pump and necessary parts. Make sure you are familiar with the pump, its parts and how it works prior to leaving the hospital. The lactation nurses should be able to help with this. Consider investing in a hands-free, breast-

pumping bra. These bras free up your hands, allowing you to multitask while you pump.

Chapter 2: Vaginal Bleeding

I t is normal to have bleeding like a period or heavier and even passing small clots (dime to quarter size off and on) for the first 5-7 days after delivery. Initially, the bleeding can be dark red to bright red in color. The color will change over time. Usually by 3-4 days postpartum, the bleeding will change to brown in color and then yellowish by about 7-14 days postpartum. Some women will continue to have intermittent spotting to light bleeding for 3-4 weeks after delivery. If you are breast-feeding, you will notice that your bleeding may increase after feedings for the first few days after delivery as the uterus contracts in response to the hormones your body is naturally producing while breast-feeding.

How to manage at home:

1.   Use pads only for the first six weeks after delivery.   Change your pads often. Avoid tampons. Tampons will not only cause trauma to an already fragile vagina, but it can also increase the risks for infection and damage any stitches placed by your physician after delivery.

2. If your bleeding seems heavier than you expect, start documenting how often you are changing your pads and how saturated they are. In addition, if you are passing clots, write down how often and how large they appear.

3.   Be patient with the process. The bleeding will stop on its own over time as the lining of the uterus sheds. There is nothing special you should do to speed up the process.

When to Call Your Doctor:

1. If you are soaking a pad in an hour or more you should call your doctor immediately.

2. If you are passing large clots (golf ball size or larger), you should call your doctor immediately.

3. If you are feeling lightheaded, dizzy, like you are going to pass out, or if your heart is racing, you should call your doctor immediately.

4. If you have a fever greater than 100.4 and heavy bleeding, you should call your doctor.

Chapter 3: Uterine Cramping

This will feel like strong period-like cramps that you may feel in your lower belly, in your back or both. Uterine cramping can be pretty intense; in fact, some women report their cramping to be as strong as contractions. This is completely normal. If you are breast-feeding, you will notice that the cramping intensifies during and after breast-feeding because the hormone released by your brain for milk let down also causes the uterus to contract. This cramping will become less and less intense over the first 72 hours after delivery and then usually resolves within five days after delivery.

How to manage at home:

1. Ibuprofen 400mg -600mg every 4-6 hours (taken with food) works extremely well for cramping. Tylenol also works well for mild to moderate pain; however, I have found ibuprofen superior for treating uterine cramping.

2. Warm compress to lower abdomen and/or lower back can help to ease cramping.

When to Call Your Doctor:

1. Constant cramping that is worsening in intensity instead of improving.

2. Nausea/vomiting associated with the cramping.

3. Fever of 100.4 or greater in addition to cramping.

4. Heavy bleeding with cramping, such as soaking through more than one pad per hour or passing clots golf ball size or larger.

Chapter 4: Vaginal Odor

It is completely normal to have a vaginal odor after your delivery. Most women will describe the odor as a metallic scent. This odor is due to the blood collecting in the vagina and mixing with the old lining of the vaginal walls. The odor will resolve on its own over time as your vaginal bleeding stops.

How to Manage at Home:

1. Clean the outer vagina with a peri-bottle. Fill the peri-bottle with lukewarm tap water and spray your bottom after you urinate, have a bowel movement and when you take a shower.

2. Sitz baths – Purchase a sitz bath basin online or at a medical supply store. Fill with two to three inches of warm (not hot) tap water and soak your bottom for up to 15 minutes, two to three times a day. Do not place soap, bath salts or bubble bath in the sitz bath, as these products can be irritating to your bottom.

3. Absolutely **avoid douching** as this can increase the risk for infection.

When to Call Your Doctor:

1. If the vaginal odor does not improve when your vaginal bleeding stops, you should notify your physician.

2. If the odor suddenly changes, you should notify your physician.

3. If you suddenly start to have vaginal itching or vaginal burning in combination with vaginal odor, notify your physician.

Chapter 5: Swelling

It is completely normal to have swelling in your legs, ankles, feet and even your labia after delivery. In fact, the swelling often worsens the first 24-48 hours after delivery and then slowly starts to improve. The extra fluid eventually gets absorbed back into your blood stream and you will urinate all the fluid out, so you may notice you are voiding more frequently over the first seven days. The swelling will completely resolve within 10-14 days after delivery.

How to Manage at Home:

1. Stay well hydrated throughout the day. Make sure you are drinking ample amounts of water (not soda

or juice) daily, approximately 64 ounces (eight, 8-ounce glasses of water). If you are breast-feeding, you should be drinking more than 64 ounces throughout the day.

2. Stay active. Walk around the house throughout the day.

3. Compression stockings can help but are not a necessity. I would recommend thigh high stockings instead of knee high stockings. You can order these online or pick them up at a medical supply store.

4. For labial swelling you can apply ice packs to your bottom. In addition, try to avoid sitting straight up and down on your bottom for long periods of time as gravity will draw fluid down into your pelvis, worsening the swelling.

5. Do not sit for long periods of time with your feet dangling down from a chair or couch. Gravity will pull all extra fluid down to your lower legs and the swelling will worsen. Instead, when you are resting, keep your legs elevated.

When to Call Your Doctor:

1. If you are having new onset headaches or visual changes in addition to worsening swelling, then you should notify your physician immediately.

2. If you have high blood pressures at home, you need to notify your physician. If the top number on the blood pressure reading is 140 or higher, or if the bottom number on the blood pressure reading is 90 or higher or both then this is considered abnormally high blood pressure and should be further evaluated by your physician.

3. If your swelling is worsening and not improving over time, you should notify your physician.

4. If you have sudden onset of pain with the swelling, then you should notify your physician.

5. If you notice that one leg is significantly more swollen than the other, notify your physician.

6. If you are having pain in your calf (that may worsen with walking), notify your physician.

7. If you have chest pain or shortness of breath, you should contact your physician.

Chapter 6: Night Sweats

You may notice during the first few nights after delivery you are waking up in the middle of the night drenched in sweat. No, you are not going through menopause and odds are you are not sick. The night sweats are a result of your rapidly changing hormones after delivery. As the hormones change, your internal thermostat has to reset itself. Night sweats will resolve within the first week after delivery.

How to Manage at Home:

1. Turn your AC down at night. Let your partner and family know that they will need extra blankets at night.

2. Keep a fan by your bed.

When to Call Your Doctor:

1. If you have a fever of 100.4 degrees or greater throughout the day or night, you should contact your physician.

2. If the night sweats continue beyond seven days after delivery, you should contact your physician.

Chapter 7: Urinary Problems

1. **Burning with urination:** Burning with urination is very common the first 48-72 hours after delivery. Try to note when you are experiencing the burning. Do you notice burning before you urinate, once you have started urinating, or when the urine hits the skin? Burning BEFORE urination may be caused by bladder spasms. If you had a foley catheter during labor, the bladder walls may become temporarily irritable and the muscle may spasm for a short time after the catheter is removed. In addition, as the baby moves through

the birth canal during vaginal delivery the bladder muscle can be irritated leading it to spasm later. Burning DURING urination may be a result of irritation of the urethra (this is the tube that carries urine from the bladder out). Burning when the urine touches the skin is usually due to vaginal tears or an episiotomy. As urine passes over these areas it can cause a stinging sensation. No matter the cause, burning with urination should resolve quickly, usually by three to four days after your delivery the pain will be gone.

How to Manage at Home:

1. Stay hydrated (with water, not soda or juice). Concentrated urine due to lack of hydration can cause more burning.

2. Use a peri-bottle during urination – Prior to voiding, fill a peri-bottle with lukewarm or cool tap water. As you start urinating, spray the water along your bottom to help dilute the urine. After you are done voiding, use

the remainder of the water in the peri-bottle to cleanse your bottom and then PAT dry (do not rub or wipe) with a clean dry towel or you can use a hair dryer on the cold setting to air dry.

3. Sitz bath – Fill a sitz bath basin with 2-3 inches of warm water and soak your bottom for five to 10 minutes after voiding. Once complete, use a clean, dry towel to PAT dry (do not rub or wipe) or use the hair dryer on the cold setting to air dry. Avoid placing soaps, bubble baths or salts in the sitz bath.

When to Call Your Doctor:

1. If the burning pain PRIOR to voiding continues beyond about 48 hours after delivery, or it seems to be worsening over time.

2. If the burning pain during or after urination does not resolve by five days after delivery or it seems to be worsening over time.

3. If you are passing only blood when you urinate (see the following entry on bloody urine).

2. Bloody urine: You will notice some blood in your urine after delivery. You may even notice small blood clots. This blood is usually coming from the vagina and not the bladder or urethra. You should notice that the amount of blood you see after urination becomes lighter and less as your vaginal bleeding improves.

How to Manage at Home: There is really not much you can do for this. It will improve as your vaginal bleeding resolves after your delivery.

When to Call Your Doctor:

1. If you are passing only blood with urination and there does not seem to be much urine, then you should notify your physician immediately.

2. If you are no longer having vaginal bleeding or spotting, but you continue to have bleeding with urination, then you need to notify your physician.

3.   If you are having worsening pain PRIOR to urination in combination with blood in your urine, then you should notify your physician.

4. If you are having middle back pain that wraps around to your side in addition to blood in your urine, then you should notify your physician.

3.   Leaking urine (stress urinary incontinence): Many women will experience some leaking of urine after a vaginal delivery. Particularly, you may notice leaking when you cough, laugh, sneeze, or exercise (jump, run, speed walk). This can be frustrating and often embarrassing. This is due to the weakening of the muscles surrounding the urethra (the tube carrying urine from the bladder out) and changes in the pelvis to accommodate the delivery of the baby.

How to Manage at Home:

1. Empty your bladder frequently. Do not wait until you can't hold your urine any longer before using the restroom. Try voiding every three to four hours whether you feel the urge to urinate or not.

2. Empty your bladder prior to exercising.

3. Kegel exercises – You can strengthen the muscles surrounding the urethra by squeezing them as if you are attempting to stop your urine stream. Hold this for five seconds and then release. You can perform this exercise anytime, anywhere (no one can tell you are doing them!). You will need to do this exercise at least 50-100 times a day to achieve results. Just like exercising to lose that baby weight, you will not see results immediately, but if you are diligent you should notice some improvement in about six to eight weeks.

When to Call Your Doctor: While, a leaking bladder will not cause physical harm, it can be psychologically stressful. If the Kegel exercises are not helping, let your doctor know. There are physical therapists that are specifically trained in pelvic floor dysfunction to help with urinary leaking. There are also surgical procedures that are available to fix this problem, however I would not recommend the surgical route unless you are done having children.

Chapter 8: Normal Aches and Pains after a Vaginal Delivery

You did it! Congratulations, you delivered vaginally! Even though vaginal delivery is the preferred mode of delivery, it does not come without its own aches and pains. After all, you just passed a cantaloupe through an opening the size of a tennis ball, so obviously there was a lot of pulling, stretching and tearing. This leads to discomfort after delivery that is often described as dull aching, throbbing or a "bruised" feeling. The purpose of this chapter is to present what is normal after a vaginal delivery and at what point you should call your doctor.

1. **Rectal pain and vaginal pain**: It may feel like pressure, almost like the baby is still there pressing down on your pelvis. The pressure feeling will improve within 48-72 hours. The "bruised" feeling may last for seven to 10 days but should improve gradually every day.

How to manage at home:

-Apply ice packs to your bottom for no longer than 20 minutes at a time, three to four times per day for the first 48-72 hours after delivery. Unless you are using an ice pack created out of a diaper, remember to lightly wrap the ice packs prior to placing against the skin.

-Try warm sitz baths twice daily for relief. Fill a small basin with two to three inches of warm (not hot) water to soak your bottom for up to 15 minutes, two to three times a day.

-Ibuprofen 400mg - 600mg every four to six hours taken with food or Tylenol 650mg every four to six hours will help to relieve this type of pain.

When to Call Your Doctor:

1. If you notice the pain is worsening over time instead of improving, you should notify your doctor.

2. If you have sudden onset of pain that is not relieved with pain medication, you should notify your doctor

3. If you are unable to sit down due to pain, you should notify your doctor.

2. **Pubic symphysis pain**: Your pubic symphysis is the bony structure in the front of your pelvis, right where your bladder is located in your lower belly. A ligament (think: a thick rubber-band between your pelvic bones) connects and holds the two bones of

your pelvis together. During pregnancy and delivery that ligament loosens up and stretches allowing the pelvic bones to separate and provide more room for the baby to move through the birth canal. After delivery this weakness of the ligament and the movement of the pelvic bones can cause pain, especially with walking. You may notice pain that can be significant at times, right in the center of your bones. This is normal and should improve over time but may take weeks to months to completely resolve.

How to manage at home:

1. Ibuprofen 400mg – 600mg every 4-6 hours or Tylenol 650mg every 4-6 hours to manage discomfort and to decrease inflammation.

2. Stay active with light activity. Walking is a great option. Yoga and Pilates allow for gentle stretching and core muscle strengthening.

3. Avoid intense activity for the first seven days after delivery (i.e., running, aerobics, stair climbing, Cross Fit).

When to Call Your Doctor:

1. If the pain is not improving over the course of a week. It may not be completely resolved within a week's time, but it should improve day by day.

2. If the pain suddenly worsens.

3. If you are unable to walk or bear weight due to pain.

4. If you feel unstable when you walk.

Chapter 9: Vaginal Tear/Episiotomy Care

V aginal tears occur commonly during childbirth due to the excessive stretching of the vaginal tissue as the baby's head and shoulders move through the birth canal and out of the vaginal opening. No vaginal tear is completely preventable. There are four different types of tears. First- and second-degree vaginal tears are the most common. In general, first- and second-degree vaginal tears are minor tears and heal well with no long-term complications. A third-degree vaginal tear is more significant because it is a tear into the anal sphincter muscle, which is the muscle that prevents stool from spontaneously leaking out of your rectum. A fourth-degree vaginal tear is the most significant tear because it is a tear through the vagina, the anal sphincter and into the rectum. Sometimes third- and fourth-degree vaginal tears don't heal well and can cause long-term complications. Luckily, third- and fourth-degree vaginal tears are rare.

An episiotomy is a small cut at the opening of the vagina your physician may have purposefully created at the time of delivery to help make room for the baby's head and shoulders. Your physician will stitch the vaginal tear (or tears) or episiotomy closed after delivery. The stitches your physician uses will dissolve within six to eight weeks after delivery.

    1. It is important to keep ALL objects out of the vagina for at least six weeks after delivery (this includes fingers, tampons, toys, etc.) to allow for the tissue to completely heal and the stitches to dissolve. If you have intercourse prior to six weeks you run the risk of

disrupting the stitches and increasing the chance for infection.

2. Keep the external vaginal tissue clean by using a peri-bottle. Fill a peri-bottle with lukewarm tap water and spray your bottom (do not place the mouth of the bottle inside the vaginal canal) after voiding and bowel movements, as well as in the shower. You do not need to use soap. Soap can be irritating and drying to the sensitive tissue of the vagina. After cleaning, pat your bottom dry with a clean, dry towel or use the hair dryer on the cold setting to air-dry. Avoid wiping. Be sure to change your pads frequently

3. Use ice packs to help with pain and swelling. You can use ice packs for 15-20 minutes at a time, three to four times a day. Never, place the ice packs directly against the skin. Wrap the ice packs in a thin towel prior to placing against the skin.

4. Sitz baths – You can purchase a small basin online or at a medical supply store. Fill the basin with two to three inches of warm (not HOT) tap water and soak your

bottom for up to 15 minutes, two to three times a day. Dry your bottom by patting dry with a clean, dry towel or use the hair dryer on the cold setting to air dry. Be sure to clean your basin well with a mild soap between uses.

5. Your pain should improve little by little every day; if you have sudden onset of pain or worsening pain then you should notify your physician. This could be a sign of an infection, disruption of the stitches, or a hematoma (collection of blood) in the vaginal wall.

6. If you had a third- or fourth-degree vaginal tear it is important you take a stool softener daily to avoid large bulky stools that are difficult to pass and can place tension on the stitches. You must follow up with your physician within the first two weeks after delivery for an examination in the office to evaluate the healing process. If you ever notice stool in the vagina you need to notify your physician as soon as possible, as this is a sign of a recto-vaginal fistula, which is a connection between the rectum and the vagina that has developed due to poor

wound healing. Unfortunately, if this happens you will need surgery to repair the defect.

Chapter 10: Physical Activity After Vaginal Delivery

O ne of the benefits of a vaginal delivery is that your physical activity is not limited afterwards. You can start exercising within seven to 10 days after delivery.

1. Lifting- There is no restriction on lifting weights after delivery.

2. You can start your regular exercise routine within a week of delivery. To avoid injury and soreness, begin by restarting the exercise routine you were doing while you were pregnant before going back to your pre-pregnancy routine.

3. Avoid swimming for six weeks to allow vaginal lacerations to heal.

4. You may notice some discomfort in your pelvis/hips the first few weeks of activity after delivery as the muscles, ligaments and bones reestablish their positions. This pain will usually resolve over time. I recommend you listen to your body. Stop if a particular exercise causes pain. Give it some time and try again in several days. While it may seem like forever, you will get back to your old routine quickly.

5. If you have never exercised before, this is a great time to start! You have a new baby, why not start a new routine? The best exercise to start with is walking. Walking is cheap, easy, low impact and most importantly you can take your baby with you when you go. You can slowly build up to running over time. If you need motivation, a personal trainer or group classes are the way to go. In addition, exercise increases endorphins, which help stabilize your mood and may decrease your risk for postpartum depression.

Chapter 11: Normal Aches and Pains after a Cesarean Section

Congratulations on your new arrival! You are a trooper! You are realizing that you are stronger than you ever thought you could be. You have been through major abdominal surgery. You have a beautiful, precious gift and a scar to show for it. Obviously, recovering from a C-section is more difficult than a vaginal delivery and will require more patience with yourself. I can attest to this. I found that patience and allowing my body to heal was quite difficult. I wanted to jump up and do all the activities I was doing before I got pregnant, but the post- operative pain quickly put me in my place.

For some women the recovery from a C-section is not only physical but also emotional because a C-section is not always a planned procedure and can often be a result of an emergency. Most women envision a healthy, uncomplicated vaginal delivery, and while that is always the goal, it is not always the final outcome. Like life, delivery of a child can sometimes be very unpredictable. It is normal to have some emotional disappointment after an unplanned C-section. However, if the emotional distress of a C-section is affecting your daily activities, then you should seek help from your physician.

The purpose of this chapter is to present what is normal to feel after a cesarean delivery and at what point you should call your doctor. You can expect to experience multiple different aches and pains after your C-section. Pain after a C-section is normal; remember, it is major abdominal surgery! However, the pain should not prevent you from being able to get out of bed and move around. Lying in bed all day is not an option because it increases your risk for blood clots and pneumonia.

1. Abdominal pain – You can expect to have pain in your lower belly and pelvis that may range from a dull ache to sharp. The pain will initially worsen when you get up and move around for the first two to three days and then slowly improve day by day.

How to Manage:

1. Pain medications – Typically, you will be given Tylenol, ibuprofen and a narcotic pain medication for five to seven days to help with the pain. The idea is to have a pain level that is tolerable enough to move around. **Do not expect to be completely pain-free**, especially for the first five to seven days. Be aware that narcotic pain medication causes some women nausea and vomiting, especially when taken on an empty stomach. Your goal should be to take the lowest dose of narcotic pain

medicine, and you should wean off narcotic pain medicine as soon as tolerable. In addition, avoid taking ibuprofen on an empty stomach as well because it can irritate the lining of the stomach and cause more pain.

2. Move around as soon as possible and as often as possible. It seems counterintuitive, but the sooner you get up and move around the less pain you will have in the long run. Try to get up and walk (with the assistance of your nurse) within the first 12 hours after your surgery.

When to Call Your Doctor:

1. If your pain suddenly worsens and is not relieved with pain medication.

2. If you are experiencing a fever higher than 100.4, in addition to pain.

3. If you have nausea and vomiting that is not related to taking the narcotic pain medication.

2. Gas pain – This pain is usually felt in your upper and lower abdomen and can move around. It is usually felt as a sharp pain that comes and goes. Gas pain is caused by the slowing of your bowel's normal constant movements leading to a buildup of gas within your intestines. You can expect that your bowels will be slower to move than normal and you may not have a bowel movement prior to discharge from the hospital. In addition, narcotic pain medication slows bowel function and can worsen gas pain as well as increase the risk for constipation. Most women will have a bowel movement within the first four to five days after a C-section.

How to Manage:

1. Moving around will help with this type of pain. Walk around the hospital and home every two to three hours for 15-20 minutes while awake.

2. Anti-gas medicine helps make the gas easier to pass. Mylicon (Gas-X) is an anti-gas medicine that is sold

over the counter. Mylicon is okay to take while breast-feeding.

    3. Wean off of the narcotic pain medication as soon as possible.

When to Call Your Doctor:

    1. If you are having pain in your abdomen and you have yet to pass gas three days after your C-section, you need to notify your physician.

    2. If you are having gas pain and nausea/vomiting, you should notify your physician.

    3. If you are having gas pain and worsening bloating of your belly then you should notify your physician.

3. Incisional pain/itching– Incisional pain and itching are normal after a C-section. Incisional pain is usually described as a sharp, pulling, ripping, burning or stretching pain at the site of the scar. It is often worsened with movement, particularly when getting in and out of bed. You may also notice that the incision will begin itching as it heals. The itching may last days to weeks but will eventually resolve. Avoid scratching at the incision to prevent infections.

How to Manage:

1. For the first four to seven days after a C-section, most women will require narcotic pain medicine in addition to ibuprofen and Tylenol to manage the incisional pain. You can start weaning off narcotics about four to five days after the C-section and depend more on the ibuprofen and Tylenol for pain management.

2. Move around as soon as possible. It seems counterintuitive, but the sooner you get up and move around the less pain you will have in the long run. Try to get up and walk (with the assistance of your nurse) within the first 12 hours after your surgery.

When to Call Your Doctor:

    1. If you notice worsening pain around the incision.

    2. If you notice swelling under the incision.

    3. If you notice worsening redness around the incision.

    4. If you notice foul smelling yellow or green drainage coming for the incision (see the following for information on incisional drainage).

    5. If you notice bright red blood coming from the incision.

4. Incisional drainage: You can expect to have some drainage from your incision the first two to three days after surgery. The drainage should be clear, light pink or dark red. Normally, drainage will stop within five to seven days after your C-section.

How to manage at home:

1. Normal drainage should be allowed to drain and will stop on its own.

2. Keep the incision dry by placing a thin, unscented maxi-pad against your incision to wick away the drainage. Change the pad frequently.

When to Call the Doctor:

1. If you notice constant bright red drainage that is saturating the bandage.

2. If you have foul smelling yellow or green drainage coming from the incision.

3. If you notice worsening redness of the skin surrounding the incision in addition to yellow or green drainage from the incision you should notify your physician.

4. If you have fever greater than 100.4, in addition to drainage from the incision, you should notify your physician.

5. Skin numbness: You will notice that the skin above and below your incision, as well as the incision itself feels numb to the touch. This is completely normal. During the C-section, microscopic nerves that supply the skin are cut. These nerves will regrow eventually, but it may take over a year for the feeling to return in the skin surrounding your incision. Some people may never get full feeling back.

Chapter 12: Incisional Care After a Cesarean Section

The incision will normally look slightly swollen with some light pink color surrounding it. You may have a small amount of clear to light pink drainage from the incision for the first 48-72 hours. Your physician may have used staples (which will be removed three to seven days after your surgery) or stitches underneath the skin (which will dissolve within eight weeks after surgery) to close your incision.

1. Staples: Staples are often used to close the skin incision. The staples should be removed within seven days after your surgery. If you wait beyond about seven days, the skin will start to grow up around the staples making them more difficult to remove. Your physician may choose to remove your staples prior to you leaving the hospital or more often she will have you return to the office to have the staples removed. Staples are easily removed with minimal discomfort. You may notice that the skin around the staples is light pink to bright pink, this can be very normal and should not cause alarm unless the actual incision is red around it and/or there is green or yellow, foul smelling drainage coming from the incision.

2. Keeping the Incision Clean: Be gentle with your incision for the first two weeks as the skin is healing. Avoid the temptation to scrub the incision.

-Take **showers only** for the first 6 weeks after surgery. Avoid submerging your incision in water (i.e., avoid sitting in bathtubs, hot tubs, swimming pools, beach water, lake water).

-While in the shower allow warm water to run down over the incision. You can use a mild, non-scented soap such as Dove or Cetaphil to gently clean the incision (use your hand and not a wash cloth to avoid the temptation to scrub). Rinse well.

-After your shower is complete, dry the incision by patting it dry with a clean towel, or you can use a hair dryer on the cold setting to air-dry.

3. Keep your incision dry: If you have extra skin hanging over your C-section scar, be sure to keep the incision dry throughout the day and night. You can place a thin, unscented maxi-pad over your scar and hold the pad in place with your underwear. The pad will wick away moisture. Be sure to change the pad throughout the day.

4. Ointments/Scar creams: Avoid the temptation of using a scar reduction ointment or cream for at least the first two weeks after the surgery. Allow the skin to completely heal prior to applying any of these products. Once the skin has healed, gently massage the product into the incision line one to two times a day. Some examples of scar ointments or creams include Mederma and Bio-Oil. Results of these products vary from person to person.

5. When to Call Your Doctor:

1. You notice the redness around the incision is growing in size.

2. The pain along the incision is suddenly worsening.

3. You notice increased swelling under or around the incision.

4. You notice foul smelling yellow to green drainage coming from the incision.

5. You have a fever higher than 100.4.

6. You notice bright red blood draining from the incision.

Chapter 13: Physical Activity after Cesarean Section

You should expect to get out of the bed to a chair or to move around your hospital room within the first 12-24 hours after your surgery. From then on it is advisable to get up and walk for 10-20 minutes every two to three hours while you are awake. Once you arrive home, avoid lying around your house, which can increase your risk for complications such as blood clots and pneumonia, in addition to increasing the length of your recovery.

1. Light activity should be started immediately. Place the baby in the stroller and go for a walk down the street. Walk around the house throughout the day.

2. Avoid STRENUOUS activity for six weeks after your surgery. Some examples of strenuous activity include:

    -running

    -sports (e.g., tennis, soccer, volleyball, basketball)

    -aerobics (e.g., step aerobics, zumba, kickboxing)

    -crossfit

    -weightlifting

    -swimming

3. Avoid heavy lifting (nothing greater than 10 pounds)

4. Stairs – If you have stairs at home, you will want to limit the number of times you go up and down them daily for the first seven to 10 days to avoid aggravating the soreness and fatigue after your C-section. Choose one floor and plan on spending most of your time on that floor.

5. After six weeks and clearance by your physician, you can slowly start exercising again. Remember, you had major abdominal surgery, so take it easy for the first two

weeks. Don't expect to pick up right where you left off prior to pregnancy or even during pregnancy. Always listen to your body. If it hurts don't do it. Wait a few more days and then try again.

6. If you have never exercised before, this is a great time to start! You have a new baby, why not start a new routine? The best exercise to start with is walking. Walking is cheap, easy, low impact and most importantly you can take your baby with you when you go. You can slowly build up to running over time. If you need motivation, a personal trainer or group classes are the way to go. In addition, exercise increases endorphins, which help stabilize your mood and may decrease your risk for postpartum depression.

Chapter 14: Hemorrhoid Care

Hemorrhoids are a result of swollen blood vessels surrounding the anus. Hemorrhoids can range from a mild nuisance to extreme pain during pregnancy. Women who have never had hemorrhoids will often develop them in pregnancy due to the increased fluid in the blood stream that can get trapped in these blood vessels. Some of the signs and symptoms associated with hemorrhoids include: rectal itching, rectal pain that worsens with bowel movements, bright red bleeding with bowel movements, and firm masses protruding out of the anus. Vaginal delivery has a tendency to temporarily exacerbate hemorrhoids. Hemorrhoids will usually improve over time after delivery, however it may take 6-8 weeks to see improvement.

How to Manage at Home:

1.   Use over-the-counter hemorrhoid relief ointments, creams or pads like Preparation H, Tucks Pads, Proctofoam, or Recticare. Each medication is OK to use while breast-feeding. Each remedy contains a different ingredient; so if one option doesn't improve your symptoms, try another.

2. Take a stool softener daily to prevent large, hard stools that can inflame hemorrhoids and cause increased pain with passage. Some great examples include Colace, Miralax and Dulcolax.

3. Stay clean by using the peri-bottle filled with lukewarm water to spray your bottom after each bowel

movement then pat dry with a clean, dry towel or use a hair dryer on the cold setting to air dry.

4. Sitz baths can provide some pain relief. Fill a sitz bath basin with two to three inches of lukewarm water and soak your bottom for up to 15 minutes, two to three times daily. Avoid adding soaps, bubble baths or salts to the water. Be sure to clean the basin well with a mild soap in between uses.

5. Stay well hydrated to guard against constipation by drinking plenty of water throughout the day (a good rule of thumb is at least eight, 8-ounce glasses daily, and even more if you are breast-feeding).

6. Increase the fiber in your diet by eating more fruits and vegetables or adding a fiber supplement.

7. Donut pillows can be helpful to relieve pressure on your bottom while sitting. The pillow is literally shaped in a ring with the center hole cut out for your bottom. You can use a small pool float ring instead.

When to Call Your Doctor:

1. If your pain is worsening despite at-home remedies.

2. If you are unable to sit down due to pain.

3. If you are unable to pass a bowel movement.

4. If you are having a large amount of bleeding with bowel movements.

Chapter 15: Hair Loss

"A ahhh...I think I am going bald!!!"

"My hair is falling out in handfuls."

This is a common concern of many women in the postpartum period. Hair loss commonly begins eight to 12 weeks after delivery as your hormones begin to normalize. Our hair grows and sheds in different phases. Normally, all of your hair is not in the same phase of hair growth or shedding, so you rarely notice the loss of hair. However, during pregnancy a large amount of your hair grows in the same phase and once that hair is done growing, it will all fall out at the same time making hair loss much more noticeable. Unfortunately, you have to ride this out. Do not fear ladies, the hair will grow back over time. Currently, there is no magic pill to prevent the hair loss many women experience after delivery.

Anemia caused by low iron can make hair loss worse. So be sure to take your prenatal vitamin and iron supplement until your iron stores in your blood return to normal. Eating a healthy diet and getting good sleep will help support new hair growth. If you continue to notice significant hair loss beyond the first six months after delivery, you should discuss this with your doctor. There may be an underlying medical problem causing the hair loss.

Chapter 16: Breast-feeding/Pumping Basics

A very personal decision, breast-feeding has been studied closely and is known to be advantageous for you and your baby. However, it is a learned behavior, and not every baby will learn to do it effectively. In addition, not every woman's body lends itself to successful breast-feeding. The bottom line is, breast-feeding is hard and takes practice, but it is worth it. I found that the first two weeks of breast-feeding was harder than recovering from my C- section. There were many days that I just wanted to give up. I recommend that any woman who has made the personal decision to breast-feed stick with it for at least four weeks. You may have to take it day by day and often hour by hour the first two to three weeks, but each of those is a victory – don't give up! There are many resources available to help guide you through your breast-feeding journey (check out the resources I have listed at the end of this book). You can do it!

What to Expect the First Week:

1. The first 48-72 hours: Your body is producing colostrum, a thick, yellowish fluid that is dense with nutrients including antibodies (the infection fighting part of our immune system) to help protect your newborn baby. Colostrum is low in volume, so don't be alarmed if you are pumping and do not get much in return.

2. Days 3-7: Sometime in the first three to seven days (usually after the first 72 hours) your breasts will become firm, more swollen and often painful as your milk comes in. In addition, you may develop a low-grade temperature

(usually no higher than 100.4) during this time. It is OK to take Tylenol for this.

- In between feedings you can apply warm compresses or take warm showers to ease the discomfort.

-Gentle massage of the breasts in the shower and just prior to breast-feeding or pumping will help soften the breast.

-Feed or pump every two hours to relieve the engorgement.

-Gentle hand expression may relieve discomfort in between feeds if necessary.

Maximizing Your Breast-feeding Experience:

1. It is easy to get dehydrated when breast-feeding, so it is important that you stay well hydrated with water (not juice or soda) throughout the day. Ideally, you should aim to drink between three to four liters of water daily.

2. Protect your nipples from cracking and bleeding by ensuring that baby is latching well. In addition, use Lanolin ointment regularly. You can apply Lanolin

ointment after each feeding. You do not need to remove the ointment prior to feeding.

3. Wear a comfortable, well-fitting breast-feeding bra. Avoid tight fitting bras.

4. Employ a lactation consultant. Lactation consultants are professionals specifically trained in assisting women and their babies with breast-feeding. Most hospitals will have lactation consultants on staff. I recommend meeting with her at least twice prior to leaving the hospital. Once you are home, if you or your baby are having difficulty with breast-feeding, it is a great idea to employ a lactation consultant as soon as possible. If you wait to see if the problem will resolve on its own, you and the baby may get frustrated and be more inclined to quit. The lactation consultant will come to your home and teach you and baby techniques to make breast-feeding easier. You can refer to the International Lactation Consultant Association (www.ilca.org) to find a consultant near you, or ask your pediatrician, obstetrician or the hospital for recommendations.

Common Breast-feeding Complications:

1. **Blocked milk ducts**: This occurs when a milk duct becomes clogged with unused milk. Blocked ducts often happen when you allow the breast to become engorged.

Symptoms to Look For: A hard, tender knot in the breast.

How to Manage:

1. Try to feed or pump for a longer period of time and more frequently throughout the day.

2. Gently massage the area prior to breast-feeding or pumping.

3. Apply a warm compress or heating pad to the affected breast prior to breast-feeding or pumping.

4. Take a warm shower and massage the area in the shower.

2. **Mastitis**: occurs when a blocked milk duct becomes infected.

Symptoms to Look For:

1. Fever (greater than 100.4 F) and chills

2. Redness of the skin over the affected breast

3. Pain in a single area of the breast around where the redness is located

4. Swelling of the affected breast

5. Flu-like symptoms such as body aches

How to Manage: If you are experiencing these symptoms, you should notify your physician. Your doctor will treat you with oral antibiotics that are safe to use while breast-feeding. In addition to antibiotics, it is recommended to continue breast-feeding and pumping from the affected breast. You can also employ the same home therapies I listed for blocked milk ducts.

3. Cracked/Painful nipples: This is often the source of many women's frustration with breast-feeding and many times leads to quitting.

How to Avoid:

- Ensure that your baby is latching on well. Ask a lactation consultant to observe your breast-feeding techniques prior to leaving the hospital to confirm baby is latching well.

- Apply Lanolin ointment after each breast-feeding session.

-Nipple shields can be used to avoid pain in women who have flat and or inverted nipples.

4. **Milk blister (milk bleb):** A milk blister occurs when milk gets trapped just under the surface of the nipple. It will appear as a small, white blister on the nipple. The blister will be painful to touch.

How to manage at home: Apply a warm, moist compress (a warm towel) to the nipple. Be sure that the towel is not hot enough to burn. Allow your baby to nurse from the affected breast after 15 minutes of warm compress. The baby's sucking action should be strong enough to open the milk blister and allow the milk to drain. If this does not work, contact your physician. Your doctor will use a sterile needle to open the milk blister and allow it to drain.

5. **Yeast infections**: Yes, you can get yeast infection of the breast/nipples. If your baby has thrush, be aware that you may get a yeast infection of the breast/nipples.

Symptoms to Look for: Most women will experience sharp shooting pains when the baby feeds. My patients have described this to me as "razor blades slicing through my breast." The skin of the breast will usually look completely normal with no redness or rashes.

Management: Notify your doctor of your symptoms. He or she will treat you with an oral anti-yeast medication. You will also need to notify your baby's pediatrician, as baby will most likely need treatment, too.

Chapter 17: Formula Feeding Basics

The decision to formula feed your baby is a personal one that is based on what is best for you and your family. Remember that this is YOUR choice. Do not allow family, friends, strangers, or the media to make you feel guilty for this decision. I have worked with many women who feel like they are bad mothers or failures because they chose to formula feed or for whatever reason were unable to breastfeed. If you are formula feeding, you are an amazing mother. You are nourishing your baby every day. While I encourage every woman to give breast-feeding a good try, ultimately, a fed baby is always best. Whatever you have to do to nourish your baby is the right thing to do. If formula feeding is a source of stress for you, seek out other mothers who are formula feeding and share stories, or talk to your physician.

What to Do With Your Breast: There are no approved medicines to "dry up" your milk.

1. Start by wearing a snuggly fitting but comfortable bra throughout the day and night.

2. Minimize stimulation of your nipples. Stimulating your nipples by rubbing them or squeezing them will send a message to your brain to tell your breast to produce milk, which will cause engorgement.

3. Place ice packs against the breast for 10-15 minutes 3-4 times a day for the first few days.

-Avoid placing ice packs directly against the skin. Instead, wrap the ice packs in a thin towel prior to placing against the breast.

Chapter 18: Your Mood

"I feel like I am losing my mind. I just start crying in the middle of a commercial and I can't explain why."

I have heard this comment or some variation of it from many of my patients. Mood changes are extremely common after delivery. Some women barely notice changes in their mood, while other women feel like they are on a roller coaster with unexpected ups and downs. Mood changes occur for several reasons:

1. Your hormones are rapidly changing after delivery

2. The new responsibility of this tiny little human who is unable to communicate his or her needs

3. Sleep deprivation

The combination of all three of these factors creates the "perfect storm" and can result in feelings of exhaustion, fear, and anxiety. These feelings can be very normal, however, if the mood changes begin to interfere with your daily living, then you should seek help.

Postpartum blues (baby blues)

Postpartum blues, also known as "baby blues," is a self-limited period of time in which women will notice changes in mood such as sadness, fear, and worry. These feelings will usually begin within three days after delivery. Postpartum blues last no longer than 14 days and should not interfere with your ability to take care of yourself or your family.

Symptoms to look for (remember these feelings should not be so strong that they take over your daily life):

1. Feelings of sadness
2. Fear
3. Anger
4. Anxiety/worry

Management of postpartum blues:

1. Get as much sleep as you can. Fatigue can worsen your symptoms. Sleep is a powerful healer both physically and mentally. The best way to accomplish this is to try to get sleep when baby sleeps. The chores can wait!

2. Seek out support from family and friends. Talk openly about your feelings. **Communication is crucial**.

3. Join a support group. Sometimes, knowing other women are dealing with the same feelings helps you to not feel isolated.

4. Set aside alone time to do something fun (even if it is only 20 minutes a day). This time alone will allow you to decompress, relax and focus on something new.

5. Exercise. Physical activity releases endorphins, which are natural mood enhancers. This can be as simple as going outside and walking for 30 minutes. You can take baby with you. Other great activities include yoga, Pilates, strength training, aerobics.

6. Find a therapist. Look for a licensed clinical social worker (LCSW) or a psychologist. These individuals are trained to help you understand your thoughts and give you exercises to help manage them. Many women find that expressing their feelings with an unbiased person is easier and more therapeutic than talking with friends or family.

Postpartum depression:

Postpartum depression is a concern when your feelings of sadness, worthlessness, and worry last longer than two weeks after delivery and/or interfere with your ability to take care of yourself or your family. Unlike baby blues, postpartum depression does not usually go away by itself without some kind of intervention.

Symptoms to look for:

1. Feelings of guilt or worthlessness

2. Uncontrollable crying

3. Change in appetite (can be eating more or less than your normal intake)

4. Lack of interest in baby, family or friends

5. Anxiety – can lead to bizarre thoughts and fears

6. Difficulty sleeping – sleeping too much or not enough

7. Poor bonding with baby

8. Thoughts of death or suicide

Management of Postpartum Depression:

1. Notify your physician of symptoms and schedule a visit to be seen as soon as possible (your physician will

want to discuss your symptoms and options for treatment).

2. Get as much sleep as you can. Fatigue can worsen your symptoms. Sleep is a powerful healer both physically and mentally. The best way to accomplish this is to try to get sleep when baby sleeps and to allow family and friends help take care of the baby so that you can rest. The chores can wait!

3. Seek out support from family and friends. Talk openly about your feelings. Communication is crucial.

4. Join a support group. Sometimes knowing other women are dealing with the same feelings helps you to not feel isolated.

5. Set aside alone time to do something fun (even if it is only 20 minutes a day). This time alone will allow you to decompress, relax and focus on something new.

6. Exercise. Physical activity releases endorphins, which are natural mood enhancers. This can be as simple as getting outside and walking for 30 minutes. You can

take baby with you. Other great activities include yoga, Pilates, strength training, aerobics.

7. Find a therapist. Look for a licensed clinical social worker (LCSW) or a psychologist. These individuals are trained to help you understand your thoughts and give you exercises to help manage them. Many women find that expressing their feelings with a nonbiased person is easier and more therapeutic than talking with friends or family.

Postpartum Psychosis:

Postpartum psychosis is a rare condition occurring in less than 1% of new moms. It typically begins suddenly within two weeks after delivery. If you or your family/friends notice any of the symptoms associated with postpartum psychosis, it should be taken very seriously. I cannot impress upon you enough the importance of seeking help immediately. These symptoms DO NOT get better on their own. In fact, these symptoms will worsen without help. Postpartum psychosis requires medical management under the direction of physicians.

Symptoms to look for:

1. Strange thoughts or beliefs that take over all of your thoughts
2. Seeing or hearing things that are not there
3. Having thoughts of hurting yourself or your baby
4. Hyperactivity while awake
5. Reduced need for sleep
6. Paranoid or suspicious
7. Rapid mood swings
8. Difficulty communicating with others

Chapter 19: Sleep

As a new mom, I underestimated the power of sleep. Those cute little peanuts lull you into a false since of security during your postpartum hospital stay. They sleep so soundly in their little bassinet at the hospital. But just wait, the second you get them home, game on! I figured I was so accustomed to being up in the middle of the night delivering other women's babies, that this whole up in the middle of the night feeding my own baby thing would be a cakewalk. Think again, sister. I fell into the trap of trying to do everything for my family and my new little man, and I neglected sleep to the point of utter exhaustion. My lack of sleep accumulated over time and affected my physical and mental well being. My c-section recovery took longer than it should have, and I quickly spiraled out of emotional control. It was not until my family stepped in and forced me to sleep that I was able to see how out of control I had become. While some lack of sleep during the fourth trimester is normal, if you are not cautious it can get out of hand.

Oh momma, please get some sleep. I am not talking eight hours, (but if you can do that, more power to you); I am talking two to four hours at a time. It is imperative to sleep. We know that sleep is restorative both physically and mentally. The average woman requires between seven to nine consecutive hours of sleep daily. During sleep your body does some pretty amazing things to repair all of the damage that occurred during the day and prepares you for tomorrow. During your fourth trimester, your body needs time to recover from the delivery, and if you had a cesarean section, this requires even more work on your body's part. Chronic fatigue leads to physical and emotional illness. Fatigue affects your ability to make decisions, your ability to anticipate problems and find solutions, and your patience for your environment and the individuals in your environment. A healthy well-rested mom makes for a healthy baby and family.

Obviously, if you are breast-feeding, you will not be able to get seven to eight consecutive hours of sleep, initially. You can, however, get two to three hours of sleep multiple times throughout the day, but you must make it a priority. Think of life during the first four to six weeks of your fourth trimester as survival mode. Food, sleep and caring for your newborn are your primary tasks. Everything else can be done later or by someone else. If you are bottle-feeding, getting consecutive hours of sleep is going to be a bit easier because you can delegate the task of baby feeding to other people, but you must be diligent about prioritizing sleep. Do not ever feel guilty for sleeping. Ultimately, you will be more prepared to care for your child and your family when you are well rested. Here are several suggestions to maximize sleep during the fourth trimester:

1. Optimize your sleeping conditions. Make the room you sleep in a sanctuary. The first four to eight weeks you may chose to have your little one sleep in the room with you, but you can still make the room sleep friendly for yourself.

- Try to make the room as dark as possible, especially for daytime naps. Black out shades work great and are usually inexpensive. If you are unable to get the room dark enough, try an eye mask.

- Keep the room temperature cool. Ideal sleeping temperature is 69-72 degrees Fahrenheit.

- Use the quietest room in the house for sleep. Ideally this room should be away from the hustle and bustle of the rest of the family activities.

- Invest in a white noise machine. A good white noise machine can drown out most outside noise. An inexpensive option is a floor or desk fan or a smart phone app (just be sure to put your phone on airplane mode before falling asleep).

2. Avoid the supermom syndrome. You don't have to do everything. Your ability to get everything done on little to no sleep does not define you as a momma. The chores can wait or be done by someone else. The baby can be held, quieted or entertained by someone else on occasion too. Ask for help without guilt and accept help when it is offered. I had a hard time with this at first. To my detriment, I wanted to do everything. Once I gave in and allowed

friends and family to help me, I realized I was actually better at momming than prior to the help. Many daily tasks can be outsourced to friends/family or even services. Get creative.

- Try ordering your groceries on line and having them delivered if that service is available in your area. If not, ask a friend/neighbor/family member to shop for you and help you put the items away.

-Sign up for a meal preparation kit subscription for one or two months. Have friends or family to make one or two meals a week for you during the first two months of your fourth trimester. Every little bit helps!

- Allow friends and family to clean and do laundry for you, or hire a cleaning service or maid if you have the means to do so.

- If you are breastfeeding, try allowing your partner to put the baby to bed after a feeding while you immediately go to sleep in order to maximize the amount of time you sleep.

-If you are exclusively pumping, purchase multiple pump parts so that you are not spending precious sleep time between feeds cleaning pump parts (at that rate you are pumping, feeding, cleaning and then by the time you are done it is time to pump again, it's a vicious cycle!). Allow someone else to clean and organize pump parts throughout the day.

- If you are bottle-feeding, let your partner feed the baby once or twice at night so that you can get more hours of consecutive sleep.

3. Avoid screen time for at least 30 minutes prior to sleep (this includes TVs, computers, I-pads, smart-phones, gaming devices). Screen time actually stimulates the brain making it more difficult to fall asleep. When you already have a limited time to sleep, you don't want to waste

precious minutes working against an active mind trying to fall asleep.

4. Avoid eating within one hour of sleep. Lying down just after eating increases the risks for acid reflux and that kind of pain will ruin anyone's sleep.

5. Try to develop a nighttime routine and stick with it. Our brains work best with routines. One size doesn't fit all. You will have to determine what works best for you and your family.

6. Consider hiring a night nurse once or twice a week. She will help take care of your baby at night so that both you and your partner can get sleep.

If you are having trouble sleeping because you are unable to turn your brain off, having reoccurring thoughts, or feeling anxious then you should speak with your physician.

Chapter 20: Sex After Baby

Sex after baby can be extremely intimidating. Not only do you not feel good in your own skin anymore, you are also exhausted and uncomfortable. The last thing you want to think about is sex. However, sex is an integral part of your relationship and needs to be fostered. It may seem like a huge undertaking, but it is not as difficult as it seems once you have a better understanding of your body. Whether you had a vaginal delivery or a C-section, you will experience many physical changes after having a baby that can affect your sex life. Some women will actually experience increased pleasure with intercourse due to the changes in position of the uterus, cervix and pelvic bones during pregnancy.

<u>Vaginal Dryness:</u> Vaginal dryness is extremely common after baby and is a common source of pain with intercourse. Vaginal dryness occurs because of the changes in hormones that women experience after childbirth. Your level of estrogen falls dramatically after delivery and the levels of prolactin and oxytocin increase. This change results in a menopausal like effect on the vaginal tissue leading to a decrease in lubrication of the vagina and even thinning of the tissue. Women who are breast-feeding may experience more significant vaginal dryness compared to women who are not breast-feeding because the prolactin and oxytocin hormones are even more elevated in breast-feeding women. Don't worry, though, it is short-lived and will return to normal in the coming months. So, be patient with the process. Invest in some lubrication. I like Astroglide because it does not get sticky with use. KY Jelly is another lubricant you can find in drug stores. Avoid lubricants with scents or menthols, as these can be irritating to the vaginal tissue and cause discomfort. If you are still experiencing significant vaginal pain with intercourse due to dryness despite the use of lubricants, talk to your doctor. Your physician may prescribe a short course of vaginal estrogen cream to help with this symptom.

Vaginal Pain: Whether you had a vaginal delivery

or C-section, vaginal pain with intercourse is common. It can be caused by vaginal dryness and changes in the pelvic floor associated with the delivery itself or with just being pregnant (your pelvis changes throughout the pregnancy to accommodate the growing fetus). If you had a vaginal delivery, then vaginal tears or episiotomies are also a source of discomfort. The discomfort will improve over time, however, the first few episodes of intercourse may be significantly uncomfortable for you, so talk with your partner and explain how you are feeling.

Options for management at home:

1. Try to relax prior to intercourse. Tensing up will tighten the pelvic floor muscles, which will cause pain with penetration.

2. Go slow.

3. Engage in foreplay prior to intercourse.

4. Stop if it hurts. Do not feel guilty if you have to stop the first few encounters. Over time the pain will improve.

5. Use **a lot** of lubricant and reapply as necessary.

6. Choose positions that allow you to be in control of the depth of penetration.

7. Perform Kegel exercises (Kegels) throughout the day to help strengthen the pelvic floor. Pilates can also strengthen the core and the pelvic floor.

-A Kegel exercise is performed by engaging the vaginal floor muscles in order to strengthen them over time. You can do this by tightening the muscles that you would use to stop your urinary stream and hold this for five seconds. You should perform this exercise 50-100 times a day. I know that seems like a lot of exercises, but the great thing is that you can perform this exercise anytime during the day without anyone even knowing you are doing it!

Lack of Desire: Libido is the desire for sexual activity. Libido is very complicated in women and is affected by multiple things. Most women will experience a decrease in libido after baby is born. This lack of desire is likely due to fatigue, changes in hormones, discomforts as discussed previously, and changes in body image. It is important that you communicate with your partner about your feelings. I recommend you remind your partner regularly that your lack of desire does not stem from lack of attraction to him or her, but the changes that have occurred all at once, which will take some time to work out.

Changes in Hormones: After delivery, your levels of estrogen fall drastically and your levels of prolactin and oxytocin increase, especially if you are breast-feeding. This basically results in a menopausal like state for the first two to three months. This leads to vaginal dryness and reduced libido.

Changes in Body Image: Many women avoid intercourse after baby because they no longer feel sexy. A deflated belly lending itself to sagging skin and stretch marks, in combination with extra weight everywhere else does not make a girl feel sexy. Believe it or not, your significant other will look past all of these changes to see a beautiful, strong woman and mother of his or her child, which adds a new type of sex appeal.

How to manage your libido at home:

1. Be honest and open with your partner – let your partner know that your lack of desire is not a result of lack of attraction to him/her (you may have to remind your partner on occasion, as some partners may need frequent encouragement).

2. Don't wait until nighttime to have sex when you are at your most exhausted state. Instead, try different times during the day. Baby's naptime is a great time!

3. You don't always have to have sex. Sometimes foreplay is just enough to satisfy both you and your partner.

4. Quickies – sex doesn't have to be long and drawn out. A short episode of sex can allow you to stay in the moment.

5. Try to avoid focusing on the parts of your body you don't like and instead, focus on one or two positive qualities. If you have trouble identifying these, ask your partner and then write them down. Remind yourself of these qualities throughout the day or when you start to focus on the negatives.

6. Avoid placing pressure on each other. Keep open communication and encourage each other. Time will help if you are both patient.

<u>Pregnancy Prevention:</u> Yes, you need to

prevent pregnancy, even if you haven't had a period yet, and even if you are breast-feeding religiously. I would love to make a promise to you that if you are breast-feeding every two to three hours that you cannot get pregnant, but believe me, I have seen it happen. Unless you are ready to have "Irish twins," I recommend some type of pregnancy prevention. There are many options and your choice will depend on if you prefer short-term contraception, long-term contraception or permanent sterilization.

Contraceptive Options:

1. **Breast-feeding:**   Breast-feeding affects fertility by preventing ovulation (the release of an egg from the ovary). You must pump or nurse your baby every two to three hours around the clock for this to occur. The effects of breast-

feeding are most reliable in the first four to six months after delivery. However, this is not a 100% guarantee. I recommend another form of contraception starting six to eight weeks after delivery if another pregnancy is not wanted.

2. Condoms: We all are probably pretty familiar with these little guys.

Pros:

1. Easy to use
2. Cheap
3. Involve no hormones
4. Easy to discontinue when ready for another pregnancy

Cons:

1. Some women are allergic to latex
2. Not the most effective form of birth control
   - Condoms have approximately 30% failure rate

3. Oral contraceptive pills: Birth control pills can be started six weeks after delivery. If you are breast-feeding, your physician will choose a progesterone-only birth control pill (the "mini" pill) because birth control pills with estrogen can reduce milk supply if your supply is not already established. If you are not breast-feeding, you can start a pill that contains both estrogen and progesterone. Pills containing both estrogen and progesterone are more effective than progesterone-only pills.

    Pros:

1. Very effective form of contraception – 95-97% pregnancy prevention rate in normal users
2. Easy to use. One pill a day.
3. Normally well-tolerated

    Cons:

1. Contains hormones – some women prefer to avoid hormones

2. Women taking progesterone-only pills must take the pill at the SAME time every day or you run a higher risk of failure

   -In contrast, pills containing both estrogen and progesterone are a little more forgiving and do not require taking the pill at the EXACT same time every day

3. You must remember to take a pill on a daily basis, which can often be very difficult to do when you are busy tending to your new baby's needs.

4. Depo Provera: Depo Provera is an intramuscular injection that you get every three months to prevent pregnancy. It feels like getting a flu shot. It is very effective at preventing pregnancy because it is easy to use and does not require you to remember to take a pill on a daily basis.

Pros:

1. Easy to use – one injection every three months.

2. You can get the shot before you leave the hospital.

3. It is progesterone-only, so it will not affect your breast milk supply if you are breast-feeding.

4. You do not have to remember to take a pill on a daily basis.

Cons:

1. It is a shot – some women hate shots.

2. It is a hormone.

3. It can be associated with weight gain – approximately five pounds over the course of a year.

4. Women who are at risk for depression should avoid Depo Provera because it can worsen the symptoms.

5. IUD (intrauterine device): An IUD is a little "T" shaped device that is placed in the uterus, usually at your six-week postpartum office visit or after. It is, in general, easy to place and is associated with minimal discomfort with insertion, especially after a vaginal delivery. The IUD is extremely effective in preventing pregnancy. In fact, it is known to be more effective than getting your tubes tied. However, unlike getting your tubes tied, you can reverse it easily by removing the IUD at any time. There are two different kinds of IUDs: the copper containing IUD (Paragard) or the progesterone containing IUD (of which there are three brands that vary in the length of time they are effective). The Paragard IUD does not contain any hormones and is good for 10 years once placed in the uterus. The Mirena, Kyleena, Skyla and Liletta are the brand names of the IUD containing the hormone progesterone that is secreted locally into the lining of the uterus. Mirena and Kyleena can stay in the uterus for up to five years to prevent pregnancy. Skyla and Liletta can stay in the uterus for up to three years to prevent pregnancy. All of the IUDs available are an ideal form of contraception for breast-feeding mommas.

Paragard IUD

Pros:

1. No hormones.
2. In office procedure, with no down time.
3. Very effective in preventing pregnancy.
4. Reversible – you can get pregnant within four weeks after removal.
5. Lasts up to 10 years.
6. Will not affect breast-feeding.

Cons:

1. Can cause some increased cramping and bleeding with your periods. I would not recommend this for women with heavy periods.
2. Some women initially experience bleeding in between periods.
3. Extremely rare risk of the IUD migrating out of the uterus.
4. Mild to moderate discomfort when inserted (i.e., period-like cramps). The cramping is easily treated with ibuprofen and lasts no longer than 24 hours.
5. Rare risk of pelvic infection in women with multiple sexual partners.

Progesterone IUD (Mirena, Kyleena, Skyla or Liletta)

Pros:

1. Small amount of progesterone secreted locally into the lining of the uterus.

2. Many women will experience shorter, lighter periods within the first year of use. Some women will stop having periods within a year after IUD placement. This IUD is ideal for women with a history of heavy periods.

3. Very effective in preventing pregnancy.

4. Reversible – can get pregnant within four weeks after removal.

5. Lasts 3-5 years (Skyla and Liletta are effective for three years. Mirena and Kyleena are effective for five years).

6. Will not affect breast-feeding.

Cons:

1. Contains some hormone.

2. Extremely rare risk of the IUD migrating out of the uterus.

3. Mild discomfort when inserted.

4. Small increased risk for ovarian cysts, which are not associated with an increased risk for ovarian cancer.
5. Rare risk of pelvic infection in women with multiple sexual partners.
6. Mild to moderate cramping after placement of the IUD, which is easily treated with ibuprofen and lasts no longer than 24 hours.

6. Nexplanon: Nexplanon is a small thin rod about the size of a matchstick that contains the hormone progesterone. The rod is inserted just underneath the skin in the upper inner arm under local anesthesia (injection of lidocaine underneath the skin). Insertion is done in the office and is usually very well tolerated. Nexplanon can stay in your body for up to three years. It is removed by making a small incision in the skin overlying the rod. Removal is also done in the office under local anesthetic.

7. Permanent Sterilization: There are a few forms of permanent sterilization. The purpose of each procedure is to interrupt the communication between the ovary and the uterus. Commonly, permanent sterilization procedures are performed after your six-week postpartum visit with your physician. However, women planning to have a C-section can have a tubal ligation performed at the time of the C-section. A tubal ligation does not significantly add to the length of time or the risks involved with a normal C-section.

Bilateral tubal ligation: The most common form of permanent sterilization is a bilateral tubal ligation (getting your tubes tied). If you have a vaginal delivery, this procedure is usually done after your six-week postpartum visit. It is done at a surgical center under anesthesia. It is a same day procedure, meaning you go home within four hours after the procedure is performed. The procedure itself usually takes 30-45 minutes to perform and is performed laparoscopically with a small camera through your belly button. Tubal ligation has up to a 3 to 5% failure rate over your lifetime, and if it were to fail, you are at risk for ectopic pregnancy, which is a pregnancy in the tubes.

Pros:

1. Same day procedure – you go home the same day it is performed.

2. Very effective – approximately 3-5% failure rate.

3. Minimally invasive procedure – done laparoscopically with small incisions (approximately the length of your pinky finger nail) in your belly button and lower abdomen.

4. Permanent sterilization – no pills to take, patches to wear or shots to get.

Cons:

1. Performed under general anesthesia.

2. Because the doctor is entering your abdomen there is a short period of down time. Plan for approximately five to seven days to recover.

3. Permanent – a common risk of a tubal ligation is future regret.

Essure: Another form of permanent sterilization is the Essure procedure, which involves placing titanium coils into the fallopian tubes to block the tubes. It too, is a same day procedure done under anesthesia. Some doctors have the ability to perform this procedure in the office.

Pros:

1. Same day procedure – you go home the same day. Some physicians have the ability to perform this procedure in their office.

113

2. The procedure is done through the vagina, so there is minimal discomfort after the procedure and no down time.

3. Permanent sterilization.

4. Extremely effective – approximately 3 to 5% failure rate.

Cons:

1. In order to confirm that the tubes are blocked with the coils, you must have an HSG, which is an imaging procedure done in a radiology suite approximately 6-8 weeks after the procedure.

2. The procedure involves the use of titanium coils.

3. Extremely rarely the coils can migrate out of the tubes.

4. Sometimes the coils cannot be placed if the tubes spasm during the procedure.

5. Permanent – there is a risk for future regret.

Chapter 21: Preeclampsia

P reeclampsia is a complication that occurs only during or after pregnancy. It is most commonly diagnosed during the third trimester prior to delivery, however it can often be diagnosed after delivery. Preeclampsia usually resolves within six to eight weeks after delivery. Preeclampsia can be dangerous and should be taken very seriously. Undiagnosed preeclampsia can lead to seizures and strokes. If you notice any symptoms, you should see your physician immediately.

Signs and Symptoms of Preeclampsia:

1. High blood pressure – if the top number on the blood pressure reading is 140 or greater and/or the bottom number on the blood pressure reading is greater than 90, then you need to notify your physician. Usually your doctor will have you come to the office for a blood pressure check.

2. New onset headache - If you are experiencing headaches that you did not have prior to delivery, then you should notify your physician. Your doctor will have you come to the office for a blood pressure check and to review your symptoms.

3. Belly pain in the right upper part of your belly near your right rib cage – If you are having pain in this area that is not associated with eating and does not seem to go away or seems to be getting worse, then you need to notify your physician.

Chapter 22: Postpartum Cardiomyopathy

ostpartum cardiomyopathy is an uncommon condition that occurs when the heart enlarges after delivery. When the heart is enlarged, the heart muscle can no longer pump blood as well as it should. Although the exact percentage of women affected by this condition is unknown, it is currently thought that postpartum cardiomyopathy occurs approximately in 1 in 1000 to 1 in 3000 women. Some of the symptoms associated with postpartum cardiomyopathy include shortness of breath (unable to catch your breath) especially with lying flat and with exertion, dry cough, fatigue, and/or heart palpitations. Some shortness of breath during pregnancy is normal especially with laying flat on your back, however shortness of breath in the postpartum period is NOT normal. If you notice any of these symptoms in the days to weeks after delivery, you need to see your doctor immediately. Postpartum cardiomyopathy is a dangerous complication of pregnancy and must be managed by a physician.

On-Line Resources

1. American College of Obstetrics and Gynecology – www.acog.org

2. International Lactation Consultant Association – www.ilca.org

3. La Leche League USA – www.lllusa.org

4. Drugs and Lactation Database – www.toxnet.nlm.nig.gov

Common Medications Compatible with Breast-feeding:

I have listed some commonly used medications that are compatible with breast-feeding. This list is by no means exhaustive. Prior to starting a new medication, consult with your Ob/Gyn physician or Pediatrician.

1. Pain medications:
   a. Ibuprofen
   b. Tylenol
   c. Percocet
   d. Oxycodone
   e. Lortab
   f. Toradol

   *****Medications containing narcotics such as Percocet, oxycodone, lortab (as listed above) are excreted in breast milk in small amounts and will have the same effect on the baby as it does on you. Narcotics can make the baby tired and less interested in feeding. It is important that if you are taking narcotics for pain after delivery that you have someone available to help take care of the baby after you have taken the medication.

2. Anti-nausea medications:
   a. Phenergan
   b. Zofran
   c. Compazene

3. Stool softeners:
   a. Colace
   b. Miralax
   c. Dulcolax
   d. Fiber-con
   e. Senokot

4. Antibiotics
   a. Ampicillin
   b. Augmentin
   c. Penicillin
   d. Dicloxacillin
   e. Macrobid

5. Blood pressure medications

    a. Labetelol

    b. Procardia (Adalat)

    c. Hydrochlorothiazide

    d. Methyldopa

6. Antidepressants:

    a. Prozac

    b. Zoloft

7. Blood thinners:

    a. Lovenox

    b. Heparin

AT THE TIME OF PUBLISHING THIS BOOK, THE MAKERS OF ESSURE HAVE DECIDED TO STOP SELLING THE DEVICE IN THE UNITED STATES. ACCORDING TO THE COMPANY ESSURE WILL NO LONGER BE AVAILABLE IN THE UNITED STATES AFTER DECEMBER 2018.

Made in the USA
Columbia, SC
19 June 2019